Disease

basic details on chronic disease management

Dr Walt wade

Contents

chapter1

diseaseintroduction to chronic disease

Chronic diseases are a growing concern worldwide, with an estimated 41 million deaths each year due to chronic disease associated causes. Chronic diseases are long-term, persistent medical conditions that often require ongoing treatment and management. They are often associated with older age, but can also affect people of all ages, including children and young adults. Unlike acute illnesses, such as the common cold, which have a short duration and can be easily treated, chronic diseases have a prolonged course, lasting for months or even years. These diseases generally progress slowly and symptoms may not be immediately apparent. Examples of chronic diseases include heart disease, stroke, cancer, diabetes, and arthritis. One of the main characteristics of chronic diseases is their high prevalence and significant impact on individuals, families, and communities. According to the World Health Organization (WHO), chronic diseases are responsible for 71% of all deaths globally, with cardiovascular diseases being the leading cause. In addition to causing suffering and premature death, chronic diseases also impose a heavy economic burden on individuals, health systems, and societies. The rise in chronic diseases can be attributed to various factors, including an aging population, lifestyle factors, and environmental and genetic factors. As people live longer, they are more likely to develop chronic diseases. Moreover, unhealthy lifestyles such as poor diet, physical inactivity, tobacco use, and excessive alcohol consumption have been linked to the development of chronic diseases. Environmental factors, such as air pollution, also play a role in the prevalence of these diseases. Additionally, some individuals may have a genetic predisposition to certain chronic diseases, making them more susceptible to developing them. Chronic diseases can have a profound impact on a person's quality of life. They can result in pain, disability, and limitations in daily activities, causing individuals to become dependent on others for care. These diseases not only affect physical health but also have a significant impact on mental health, with many individuals experiencing depression, anxiety, and social isolation. One of the biggest challenges in managing chronic diseases is their lifelong nature. Unlike acute illnesses, which can be treated with short-term interventions, chronic diseases require long-term management, often involving multiple healthcare providers, specialized care, and ongoing monitoring. This can be emotionally and financially taxing for patients and their families, as well as healthcare systems. Prevention and early detection are essential in mitigating the impact of chronic diseases. Adopting healthy lifestyle habits, such as balanced nutrition, regular exercise, and avoiding harmful substances, can go a long way in preventing the onset of these diseases. Additionally, early detection through regular screenings can lead to early intervention and improved outcomes. Furthermore, the management of chronic diseases requires a comprehensive, patient-centered approach that addresses not only the physical symptoms but also the psychological, emotional, and social well-being of individuals. This involves collaborative care between patients, their families, and a multidisciplinary team of healthcare professionals such as doctors, nurses, dietitians, physiotherapists, and mental health providers. The advancement of technology has also greatly benefited the management of chronic diseases. Telemedicine, for example, has allowed patients to remotely access healthcare services, reducing the burden of frequent hospital visits. Digital health tools, such as smart devices and mobile apps, have also made it easier for individuals to track their health behaviors, monitor their condition, and communicate with their healthcare providers. Despite these advancements, there are still significant barriers to the effective management of chronic diseases. These include limited access to healthcare in underserved areas, lack of patient education and awareness, and financial constraints. Additionally, healthcare systems in many countries are often not equipped to provide comprehensive and integrated care for chronic diseases, leading to fragmentation and poor coordination of services. In conclusion, chronic diseases are a global health challenge that requires urgent attention. These long-term conditions have a significant impact on individuals, families, communities, and healthcare systems. Prevention, early detection, and comprehensive and patient-centered management are key strategies in addressing the burden of chronic diseases. Moreover, there is a need for continued investment in research and policy initiatives to improve the prevention, management, and outcomes of chronic diseases.

chapter2

chronic disease list

The list of chronic diseases is extensive, as there are many different types of conditions that can fall under this category. Some of the most common chronic diseases include heart disease, cancer, diabetes, chronic obstructive pulmonary disease (COPD), and arthritis. However, there are many other chronic diseases that are less well-known but can have a significant impact on an individual's health and quality of life. One of the primary characteristics of chronic diseases is that they have no immediate cure. While some may be managed through medication or lifestyle changes, there are currently no known cures for many chronic diseases. This means that patients with chronic diseases often require ongoing medical care and must learn to manage their symptoms and condition for the rest of their lives. One of the most prevalent chronic diseases is heart disease, also known as cardiovascular disease. It refers to a range of conditions that affect the heart and its blood vessels, including high blood pressure, coronary artery disease, and heart failure. Heart disease is the leading cause of death globally, with an estimated 17.9 million deaths attributed to it in 2019 alone. Another chronic disease that affects a significant number of individuals worldwide is cancer. Cancer is a group of diseases that occur when abnormal cells in the body continue to divide and grow uncontrollably, forming a tumor. There are many different types of cancer, each with its own unique set of risk factors and treatments. It is estimated that in 2020, there were 19.3 million new cancer cases and 10 million cancer-related deaths globally. Diabetes is another chronic disease that is estimated to affect over 463 million people worldwide. Diabetes occurs when the body either cannot produce enough insulin (a hormone that regulates blood sugar levels) or cannot use the insulin it produces effectively. This leads to high levels of sugar in the blood, which can cause severe complications if not managed properly. Chronic obstructive pulmonary disease (COPD) is a group of lung diseases that make it difficult to breathe. The primary cause of COPD is long-term exposure to irritants, such as cigarette smoke or air pollution. It is the fourth leading cause of death globally, with an estimated 3.2 million deaths attributed to it in 2019. Arthritis is another chronic disease that affects a significant portion of the population, particularly the elderly. It refers to a group of over 100 different conditions that affect the joints, causing pain, stiffness, and swelling. Arthritis can also affect other parts of the body, such as the organs and eyes, and can significantly impact an individual's mobility and independence. In addition to these common chronic diseases, there are also many other conditions that fall under this category, including asthma, autoimmune diseases, AIDS, and mental health disorders like depression and anxiety. Each of these diseases has its own unique set of symptoms and treatment options. However, they all share the common characteristic of being long-term and requiring ongoing management. One of the main challenges of living with a chronic disease is the impact it can have on an individual's daily life. Chronic diseases can affect a person's physical, emotional, and mental well-being, making it challenging to perform daily tasks and maintain social connections. Patients may also experience financial strain due to the cost of medication and ongoing medical care. Chronic diseases can also lead to potential complications that can significantly impact an individual's health and quality of life. For example, individuals with heart disease may be at a higher risk of developing blood clots or having a heart attack. Similarly, diabetes can lead to severe complications such as kidney failure, blindness, and nerve damage. To manage chronic diseases effectively, it is essential to have proper medical care and support. This includes regular check-ups, medication management, and lifestyle modifications such as diet and exercise. For some chronic diseases, treatment options may also include surgery or other medical procedures. Support groups and education programs can also play a crucial role in helping individuals cope with their chronic disease. These resources provide a safe space for individuals to share their experiences and learn from others who are going through similar challenges. They also offer practical tips and tools for managing the disease and improving overall well-being.

how to prevent chronic disease

1. Maintain a healthy diet A healthy and balanced diet is essential for preventing chronic diseases. A diet rich in fruits, vegetables, whole grains, lean proteins, and healthy fats is known to reduce the risk of developing chronic diseases. These foods are packed with essential nutrients, antioxidants, and fiber, which help to protect our bodies against chronic diseases. On the other hand, a diet high in saturated fats, processed

foods, and added sugars can contribute to the development of chronic diseases, such as heart disease, diabetes, and obesity. Therefore, it is important to limit the consumption of unhealthy foods and focus on incorporating more whole, nutritious foods into our diets. 2. Engage in regular physical activity Exercise is another crucial factor in preventing chronic diseases. Being physically active can help maintain a healthy body weight, reduce the risk of heart disease, stroke, and diabetes, and improve mental health. The World Health Organization recommends at least 150 minutes of moderate intensity or 75 minutes of vigorous intensity exercise per week for adults. This can include activities such as walking, running, swimming, cycling, or any other physical activity that gets your heart rate up. By staying active, we can lower our risk of developing chronic diseases and improve our overall well-being. 3. Avoid tobacco and limit alcohol consumption Tobacco use and excessive alcohol consumption are major risk factors for chronic diseases. Smoking is responsible for one in five deaths in the United States and is a leading cause of preventable death worldwide. It increases the risk of developing lung cancer, heart disease, stroke, and respiratory diseases. Similarly, excessive alcohol consumption is linked to liver disease, heart disease, and certain types of cancer. By avoiding tobacco and limiting alcohol consumption, we can significantly reduce our risk of developing chronic diseases. 4. Get regular check-ups Regular health check-ups are essential for detecting chronic diseases at an early stage. Many chronic diseases, such as diabetes and high blood pressure, often show no symptoms in the early stages. By getting routine check-ups, we can identify these diseases and start treatment early, preventing further complications. Additionally, regular check-ups can help us keep track of our overall health and make necessary lifestyle changes to prevent chronic diseases. 5. Manage stress Chronic stress has been linked to an increased risk of many chronic diseases, including heart disease, depression, and diabetes. However, by learning to manage stress, we can reduce our risk of developing these diseases. Some effective stress management techniques include exercise, meditation, deep breathing techniques, spending time with loved ones, and practicing self-care. By finding healthy ways to cope with stress, we can improve our overall health and well-being. 6. Maintain a healthy body weight Being overweight or obese is a significant risk factor for many chronic diseases, including heart disease, stroke, and diabetes. Therefore, maintaining a healthy body weight is crucial for preventing these diseases. A balanced diet and regular physical activity are key components in maintaining a healthy weight. If you are overweight, a 5-10%

weight loss can significantly reduce your risk of developing chronic diseases. 7. Protect yourself from environmental hazards Exposure to certain environmental hazards can increase the risk of chronic diseases. For example, exposure to air pollution, chemicals, and secondhand smoke has been linked to an increased risk of heart disease, respiratory diseases, and cancer. To prevent these diseases, it is essential to protect ourselves from these hazards by wearing protective gear, such as masks and gloves, and avoiding exposure whenever possible. 8. Practice good hygiene Bacterial and viral infections can weaken our immune system and increase the risk of chronic diseases. Therefore, practicing good hygiene is crucial for preventing these infections. Some simple ways to practice good hygiene include washing your hands regularly, covering your mouth and nose when coughing or sneezing, and avoiding close contact with sick individuals. By reducing our risk of infections, we can also reduce our risk of developing chronic diseases. 9. Get vaccinated Vaccinations are a crucial component of disease prevention, especially for chronic diseases. For example, the flu vaccine significantly reduces the risk of developing flu-related complications, such as pneumonia, which can lead to chronic respiratory problems. Similarly, getting vaccinated against certain types of cancer, such as HPV, can significantly reduce our risk of developing these diseases. By staying up to date with vaccinations, we can protect ourselves from many chronic diseases. 10. Educate yourself and others Education is a powerful tool in preventing chronic diseases. By educating ourselves about the risk factors and ways to prevent chronic diseases, we can make informed decisions about our health. Additionally, by sharing this information with others, we can help prevent chronic diseases in our communities. Good sources for information include healthcare professionals, reputable websites, and educational programs.

chapter3

chronic disease management

The management of chronic diseases is typically a multidisciplinary approach that involves collaboration between patients, healthcare professionals, and support systems. The goal is to provide the most comprehensive and integrated care for patients with chronic diseases, which often have complex physiological, psychological, and social aspects. Therefore, proper management requires the adoption of a holistic and patient-centered approach that takes into account the individual needs and preferences of each patient. The first step in chronic disease management is the accurate diagnosis of the condition. This involves a thorough assessment of the patient's medical history, risk factors, and physical examination. In some cases, laboratory tests or imaging studies may be required to confirm the diagnosis. It is essential to involve the patient in this process and ensure that they understand their condition and the treatment options available. Patients must also be informed of the potential complications and the importance of adhering to the treatment plan. Once a diagnosis is made, the next step in chronic disease management is to develop an individualized treatment plan. Depending on the type of chronic disease, the treatment may involve lifestyle modifications, medication, surgery, or a combination of these. Lifestyle changes such as following a healthy diet, regular exercise, and avoiding harmful habits like smoking and excessive alcohol consumption can significantly improve the outcome of chronic diseases. Medications are also commonly used for managing chronic conditions, and regular follow-ups with healthcare professionals are necessary to monitor the patient's response and adjust the treatment accordingly. In some cases, surgery may be required to manage certain chronic diseases. For instance, coronary artery bypass surgery is often recommended for patients with severe heart disease, and joint replacement surgery may be an option for those with chronic arthritis. These procedures are generally last resorts when other treatment options have failed, and strict post-surgical care is essential to ensure optimal recovery and prevent complications. Chronic disease management also includes regular monitoring and follow-up to assess the progress of the condition and make any necessary changes in the treatment plan. This is particularly important for patients with conditions like hypertension and diabetes, where close monitoring of blood pressure and blood sugar levels is crucial for achieving good outcomes. Patients should be encouraged to keep a record of their symptoms, medication use, and any significant changes in their health. Regular follow-ups also provide an opportunity to educate patients about their condition and address any concerns or questions they may have. Patient education is a vital component of chronic disease management. Patients must have a thorough understanding of their condition, its underlying causes, and the treatment plan. This includes knowing the importance of adhering to medication regimens, following lifestyle recommendations, and recognizing any warning signs or triggers that may worsen their condition. Patients should also be aware of the benefits of self-management and informed about any support systems or resources that may help them cope with their chronic illness. In addition to medical treatments, chronic disease management also requires the support of family and caregivers. Living with a chronic disease can be challenging, and patients often rely on the emotional and practical support of their loved ones to manage their condition. Family members should be involved in the patient's care plan and educated about the disease and its management to provide adequate support when needed. Technology has also played a significant role in improving chronic disease management. The development of electronic health records, remote patient monitoring, and mobile health applications has revolutionized the way healthcare is delivered. These tools allow for better patient engagement, more efficient management of chronic conditions, and facilitate timely communication between patients and their healthcare providers. Patients also have access to a wealth of information and resources online, making it easier for them to manage their condition and actively participate in their care.

chapter4

causes of chronic disease

One of the primary causes of chronic diseases is unhealthy lifestyle habits. With the rise of modernization and urbanization, individuals are exposed to unhealthy dietary choices, a sedentary lifestyle, and increased stress levels. These lifestyle habits increase the risk of developing chronic diseases such as obesity, type 2 diabetes, and heart disease. Consuming a diet high in processed and fast foods that are high in calories, sugar, and unhealthy fats can lead to weight gain and an increased risk of chronic diseases. Additionally, a sedentary lifestyle with minimal physical activity can also contribute to obesity and its associated health problems. Lack of physical activity can lead to a slower metabolism, muscle loss, and increased body fat, all of which are risk factors for chronic diseases. Moreover, stress can also play a significant role in the development of chronic diseases as it contributes to unhealthy lifestyle habits, such as overeating, smoking, and excessive alcohol consumption. Genetics also play a crucial role in the development of chronic diseases. While not all diseases have a genetic component, some individuals may have a predisposition to certain conditions, making them more susceptible to developing these diseases. For example, individuals with a family history of heart disease or diabetes are at a higher risk of developing the same condition. Genetic factors can also influence an individual's response to certain lifestyle habits, such as diet and exercise, and can determine their susceptibility to chronic diseases. Although genetics cannot be controlled, individuals can be aware of their family history and take proactive measures to reduce their risk, such as maintaining a healthy lifestyle and getting regular health check-ups. Environmental factors can also contribute to the development of chronic diseases. Air pollution, exposure to toxins and chemicals, and inadequate access to clean water can all have long-term effects on an individual's health. Air pollution can cause respiratory diseases, while exposure to toxins and chemicals, such as those found in pesticides and industrial products, can lead to various types of cancer. Inadequate access to clean water can also result in the spread of water-borne diseases, causing chronic health problems. Additionally, environmental factors can also impact an individual's mental health, which can contribute to the development of chronic diseases. Poor living conditions, high levels of stress, and lack of access to healthcare can all impact an individual's mental wellbeing, which in turn can lead to chronic health problems. Another significant cause of chronic diseases is the ageing population. With advances in modern medicine and technology, the average lifespan has increased globally. However, as individuals age, their bodies become more vulnerable to chronic diseases. The body's natural ability to repair and regenerate damaged cells and tissues decreases with age, resulting in a higher susceptibility to various medical conditions. Moreover, age-related chronic diseases often lead to further health complications, making them more challenging to manage and control. Some chronic diseases are also caused by infectious agents, such as viruses, bacteria, and parasites. For example, chronic hepatitis B and C are caused by infection with the hepatitis B or C virus. These infections can lead to chronic liver disease, liver cancer, and other serious health problems. Additionally, chronic diseases such as pneumonia and tuberculosis are caused by bacteria and can result in severe respiratory conditions if left untreated. Social and economic factors also play a significant role in the development of chronic diseases. Low-income individuals and those living in impoverished areas are at a higher risk of developing chronic diseases due to the lack of access to healthcare, basic resources, and education. These factors can also contribute to poor lifestyle choices, such as a poor diet and lack of physical activity, which can lead to chronic diseases. Furthermore, individuals from marginalized communities and minority groups may also face systemic discrimination and barriers to healthcare, increasing their risk of developing chronic diseases.

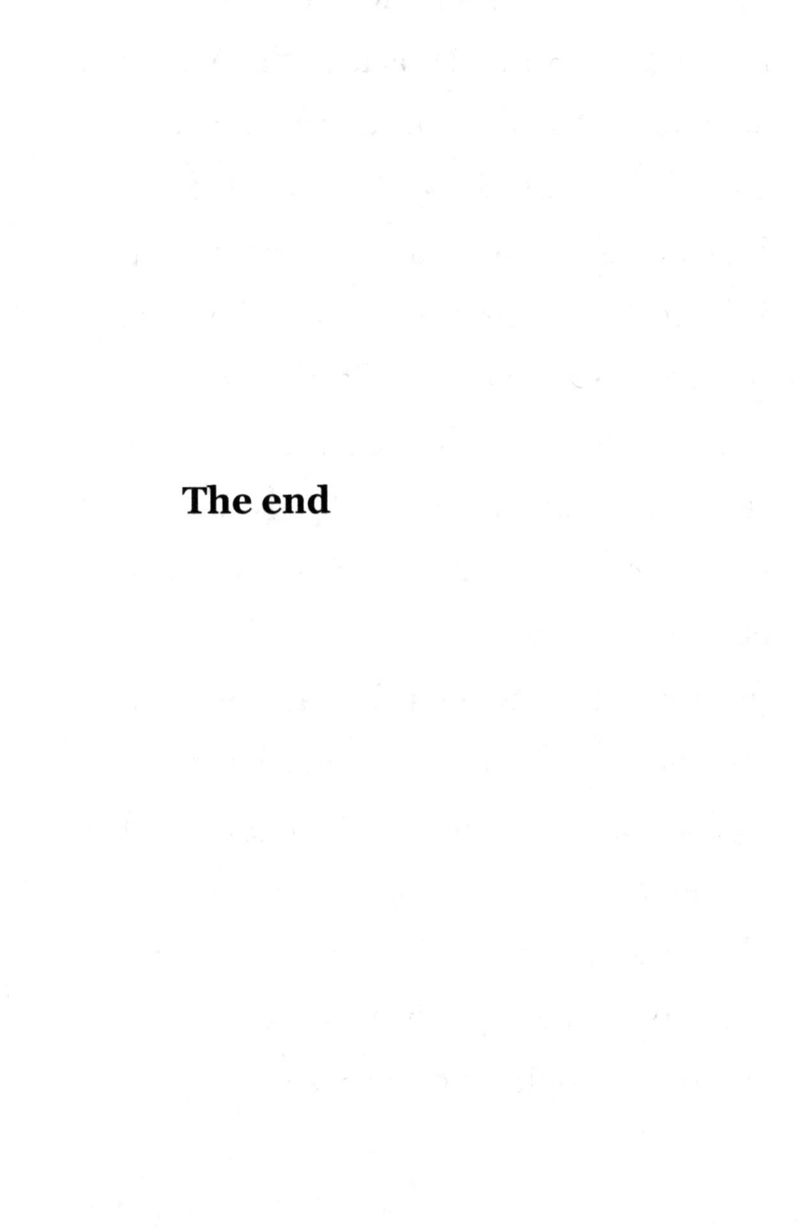

The end

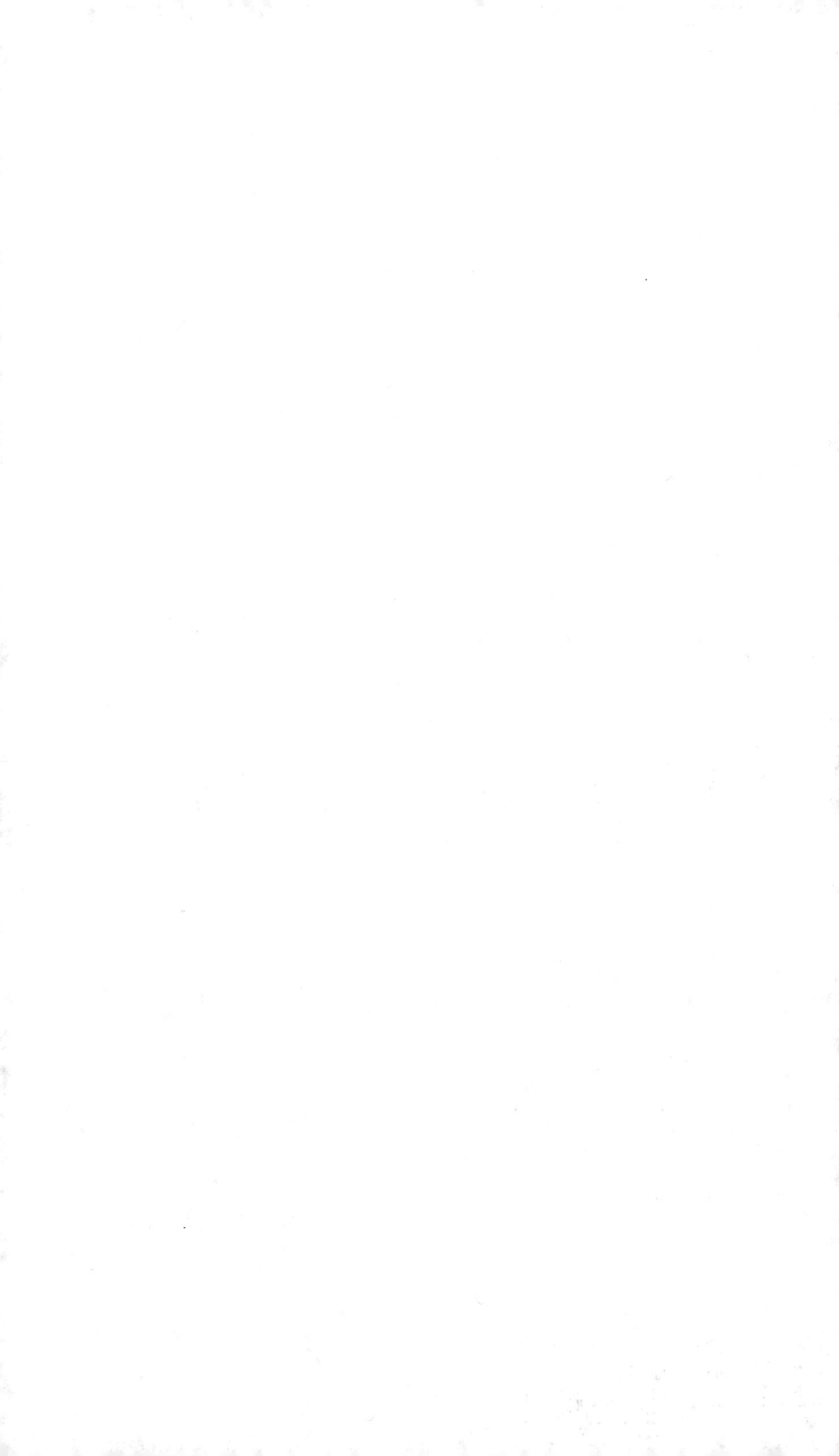